Joanna

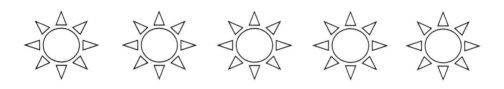

# The Power
# of
# Vitamin B

DL Publishing

# Free Educational Video!
# Visit
# http://lapappaorganics.com

## Watch the video for educational highlights

## The Power of Vitamin B

## Copyright © 2017 by Joanna Shanti

Published and Distributed Worldwide by:

DL Publishing
dlazur.com

# Dedication

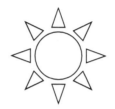

I dedicate this book to all of you seeking to find that missing link to designing a healthy and happy life.

Big thanks to all of the wonderful people who made this book possible Roger, DL Publishing Staff, and Oana.

# Table of Contents

# 1. What is Methylcobalamin?

Methylcobalamin is a cobalamin, which is a form of vitamin B12. Cobalamins are similar to hemoglobin, except that instead of iron they contain cobalt. In order to understand what methylcobalamin is, you first need to learn a couple of basic things about vitamin B12 and cobalamins. Vitamin B12 is very important for the mental and physical health, and this is why you need to know how it occurs in nature and how it is synthetized in order to be used in pharmaceutical products. This is the only guarantee that you will make an informed decision when you choose to take vitamin B12. The fact that vitamin B12 has four different types is of crucial importance, because each type is produced in a certain way, and has certain effects on the human body.

Vitamin B12 is a water-soluble vitamin with a key role in the normal functioning of the brain and nervous system, and in the formation of blood. It is one of the eight B vitamins, and it was discovered from its relationship to pernicious anemia, which is an autoimmune disease caused by the destruction of the intrinsic factor in the stomach. The intrinsic factor is a protein that ensures a normal absorption of B12. The lack of intrinsic factor causes a vitamin B12 deficiency.

Vitamin B12 mediates two principal enzymatic pathways: the methylation process of homocysteine to methionine, and the conversion of methylmalonyl coenzyme A (CoA) to succinyl-CoA. As a co-factor, B12 facilitates the methylation of homocysteine to methionine, which is later activated into S-adenosylmethionine (SAM-e) which donates its methyl group to methyl acceptors such as myelin, neurotransmitters, and membrane phospholipids.

Vitamin B12 is the largest and most structurally complicated vitamin, and it is produced by bacteria, including bacteria which are found in human and animal intestines. Industrially, it can be produced only through bacterial fermentation-synthesis. It has four different forms: cyanocobalamin, hydroxocobalamin, methylcobalamin, and adenosylcobalamin.

Cyanocobalamin is an artifact formed from using activated charcoal, which always contains trace cyanide, to purify hydroxocobalamin. Hydroxocobalamin is a medicinal form of vitamin B12 produced by bacteria, and the two naturally occurring forms of B12 in the human body are adenosylcobalamin (the cofactor of Methylmalonyl Coenzyme A mutase) and methylcobalamin (the cofactor of enzyme Methionine synthase), which the human organism produces by converting different forms of the vitamin. While cyanocobalamin is the most commonly used form of cobalamin because it is easier and cheaper to produce, methylcobalamin is obviously the healthiest and most efficient one.

Methylcobalamin features an octahedral cobalt (III) center, and it can be obtained as bright red crystals. It is a rare example of a compound that contains metal-alkyl bonds. Physiologically, it is equivalent to vitamin B12, and it can be used to prevent or treat pernicious anemia.

Methylcobalamin is considered the most potent form of Vitamin B12 found in nature because the body can assimilate it directly, without having to go through different processes to first make it "body friendly". This is due to the fact that it actually produces it. It is the only cobalamin that has the ability to activate the methionine/homocysteine biochemical pathway directly, a pathway which is responsible for the body's entire sulfur-based detoxification system and the formation of S-adenosylmethionine (SAM-e) – the universal methyl donor.

Methylcobalamin can be produced in the laboratory by reducing cyanocobalamin with sodium borohydride in alkaline solution, followed by the addition of methyl iodide.

# 2. Cyanocobalamin vs. Methylcobalamin

The main difference between cyanocobalamin and methylcobalamin is the fact that the first one is entirely artificial, while the second one occurs naturally. Also, while methylcobalamin contains a methyl group, cyanocobalamin contains a cyanide group. The reason for which cyanocobalamin is considered a form of vitamin B12 is that the body can convert it to any one of the active B12 compounds, such a methylcobalamin. However, it is largely artificial, and one of its worst effects is that it leaves a cyanide residue in the blood stream. Cyanide is a highly poisonous toxin which the body cannot break down on its own, and which you do not want in your system. Conventional medical providers argue that the cyanide is safe and alternative providers advise that a complete detox is needed to remove it.

Cyanocobalamin is the most air-stable of the B12 forms. It is the easiest to crystallize and, therefore, easiest to purify after it is produced by bacterial fermentation, or synthesized in vitro. In short, this is how cyanocobalamin is produced:

A variety of microorganisms are fermented, and the result is a mixture of methylcobalamin, hydroxocobalamin, and adenosylcobalamin. This mixture is converted to cyanocobalamin by adding potassium cyanide in the presence of sodium nitrite and heat. Because hydroxocobalamin has a great affinity for cyanide, activated charcoal is used to purify it. Naturally, activated charcoal contains cyanide, which hydroxocobalamin picks up, and is thus changed into cyanocobalamin. Cyanocobalamin is used in most pharmaceutical preparations exactly because the cyanide it contains stabilized the molecule.

However, this form of vitamin B12 can have several side effects due to the cyanide residue it leaves in the organism. Some patients may have allergic reactions, such as hives, while others may experience headache, nausea, stomach upset, or diarrhea. Even though the cyanide that is liberated in the organism when the body converts cyanocobalamin into methylcobalamin is very small and its toxicity is negligible, it is good to know that you will need to go through a complete detox if you want to make sure you get the toxin out of your system.

Cyanocobalamin is safe, and injectable cyanocobalamin is the most commonly injectable vitamin B12 in the United States. It has been scientifically proven to be great for energy, and it is successfully used to treat pernicious anemia, liver disease, kidney disease, thyrotoxicosis, hemorrhage, and many other illnesses. Also, it is usually prescribed to gastric bypass patients whose bodies cannot properly absorb B12 via food or vitamins because a part of their small intestine was bypassed.

Cyanocobalamin is very cost effective, and this is why most people prefer it. However, methylcobalamin is known to cure more complicated health problems with the advantage of leaving no toxins behind. Moreover, it balances the nervous system, increases weight reduction, induces better sleep, and reduces stress. It is used in the treatment of peripheral neuropathy, diabetic neuropathy, and as a preliminary treatment for amyotrophic lateral sclerosis. This is because methylcobalamin is the specific form of B12 needed for the health of the nervous system, which means that it is also an important nutrient for vision. While methylcobalamin can improve visual accommodation, it seems that cyanocobalamin is completely ineffective.

Tests have shown that methylcobalamin remains in the body for a longer period of time and at higher levels than cyanocobalamin, which means that your body is supplied with vitamin B12 for longer. Knowing all this, you can now understand why it is better to opt for methylcobalamin instead of cyanocobalamin when you want to increase your body's absorption of B12.

13

# 3. Warning Signs of Vitamin B12 Deficiency

One way to determine a vitamin B deficiency is by taking a look at the foods that you eat, since vitamin B12 works in conjunction with the other B vitamins to alleviate various illnesses and deficiencies.

Below I have listed the vitamins that work in conjunction with vitamin B12, along with the foods that contain the vitamin sources:

**Vitamin B1 (thiamine)**: Naturally occurs in kidney beans, wheat germ, peas, whole grains, and brown rice

**Vitamin B2 (riboflavin)**: Naturally occurs in brewer's yeast, kidney beans, broccoli, Brussels sprouts, asparagus, green leafy vegetables, wheat germ, almonds, cottage cheese, yogurt, tuna, and salmon.

**Vitamin B3 (niacin)**: Brewer's yeast, liver, poultry, fish, peanuts, eggs, milk, whole grains.

**Vitamin B4 (choline)**: Liver, cauliflower, broccoli, brewer's yeast, spinach, wheat germ, tofu, grapefruit, almonds, peanuts.

**Vitamin B5 (pantothenic acid)**: Liver, kidney, egg yolks, cheese, whole grain cereals, cauliflower, sweet potatoes, beans, brewer's yeast.

**Vitamin B6 (pyridoxine)**: Soybeans, poultry, tuna, bananas, legume, potatoes, oatmeal, wheat germ.

**Vitamin B7 (biotin)**: Liver, leafy green vegetables, Swiss chard, raw egg yolk.

**Vitamin B8 (inositol)**: Fruits, beans, grains, nuts.

**Vitamin B9 (folate)**: Spinach, liver, brewer's yeast, asparagus, Brussels sprouts, dairy products, poultry, meat, eggs, seafood, grains.

**Vitamin B12 (cobalamin)**: Liver, oyster, poultry, fish, eggs, dairy products.

Typically, if an individual is diagnosed with one vitamin deficiency, there is a chance that they may also have other vitamin deficiencies. For example: if you are diagnosed with low iron (anemia), then you may also have a vitamin B deficiency.

The symptoms of vitamin B12 deficiency are subtle, slow in onset, and easy to misdiagnose. They can be painful, disorienting, debilitating, and even life-threatening. Vitamin B12 plays a crucial direct or indirect role in the metabolic processes, and in the development and functioning of the blood, nerve, skeletal and cardiac muscle cells, and the brain.

Vitamin B12 deficiency is also known as hypocobalaminemia, and it typically features a low blood level of vitamin B12. The deficiency is common to all age groups and, unfortunately, it is too often diagnosed late. Neuropsychiatric symptoms can precede hematologic signs. B12 deficiency can cause permanent damage to nervous tissue if left untreated longer than 6 months.

A very common health condition that can cause B12 deficiency is pernicious anemia, which is an autoimmune disease that destroys gastric parietal cells. The destruction of these cells leads to a serious lack of intrinsic factor, which is directly responsible for the absorption of vitamin B12 from the food we consume. If untreated, both pernicious anemia and B12 deficiency can prove to be fatal.

## *Those who are at risk for B12 deficiency are:*

- Vegans and vegetarians who don't eat dairy or eggs, because vitamin B12 is found only in animal products;
- People who have problems with absorbing nutrients due to conditions such as Crohn's disease or pancreatic disease;
- People who underwent gastric bypass surgery;
- People who are infected with Helicobacter pylori, an organism in the intestines which can cause ulcer. H. pylori damages stomach cells that make intrinsic factor, thus preventing the proper absorption of B12;
- People with an eating disorder;
- The elderly.

While some symptoms of vitamin B12 deficiency are easily reversed by boosting the intake of vitamin through supplements that contain methylcobalamin, other symptoms can stay even long after your B12 levels have returned to normal. This is why it is important to pay attention to these symptoms and consult a doctor as soon as you have the slightest suspicion that you might be suffering of vitamin B12 deficiency. If it is not discovered early enough and treated appropriately, it can cause some serious, irreversible damage.

The symptoms of B12 deficiency are divided into four broad categories: hematologic, neurological, psychiatric, and cardiovascular[1].

## *Hematologic Symptoms*

---

[1] *Vitamin B12 Deficiency*, Robert C. OH, CPT, MC, USA, U.S., Army Health Clinic, Darmstadt, Germany; David L. Brown, MAJ, MC, USA, Madigan Army Medical Center, Fort Lewis, Washington; *American Family Physician.* 2003 Mar 1;67(5):979-986 (http://www.aafp.org/afp/2003/0301/p979.html).

Because vitamin B12 is essential to the proper development and functioning of red blood cells, a deficiency can cause a lack of healthy red blood cells, which results in anemia. The symptoms of anemia are weakness, fatigue, light-headedness, rapid heartbeat, rapid breathing, and pale color of the skin. It may also cause bruising or bleeding, including bleeding gums, nose bleeds, and excessive menstrual bleeding. Other symptoms include a swollen and inflamed tongue, digestive issues, such as constipation or diarrhea, and unexplained weight loss.

Usually, these are the early signs of vitamin B12 deficiency. If you treat it when you first develop some of these symptoms, you might limit or completely prevent long-lasting nerve damage.

### Neurological Symptoms

Vitamin B12 is essential to the development of healthy nerve cells because it helps maintain healthy myelin, which is a fat-rich coating that covers the nerve cells. Myelin helps to insulate each cell, and a healthy myelin coating allows your nerves to send rapid electrochemical signals to neighboring cells. If your myelin becomes damaged and starts to break down, your nerves no longer communicate properly, and you see a decrease in nervous system function.

Symptoms that warn you that the deficiency has started to affect the nervous system include tingling, numbness or unexplained pain in the fingers and toes, impaired perception of deep touch, and difficulty walking. Also, lack of proper nerve functioning can cause muscle wasting, and in time, the muscles controlling the sphincters of the iris, stomach, small intestine, gall bladder, anus and others might no longer function as designed.

### Psychiatric Symptoms

These symptoms are strongly connected to the neurological ones because, naturally, the malfunctioning of the nerve cells extends to the brain and its psychological functions. Thus, you might experience mood changes, irritability, depression, memory loss, disorientation, and, in severe cases, dementia.

For example, depression is not always recognized as a vitamin B12 deficiency, but you need to know that many people manifest depression which was actually initiated by a vitamin B12 deficiency.

### Cardiovascular Symptoms

B12 deficiency has been linked to hyperhomocysteinemia, or high blood homocysteine levels. This is associated with the breakdown of the red blood cells, which increases the risk of blood clots, heart attacks and strokes. It is an independent risk factor for atherosclerotic disease.

Vitamin B12 deficiency can cause severe and irreversible damage, especially to the brain and nervous system. These symptoms of neuronal damage may not reverse after correction of hematological abnormalities, and the chance of complete reversal decreases with the length of time the neurological symptoms have been present.

I am currently researching a hypothesis that women who are diagnosed with low iron and vitamin B levels during pregnancy, and continue the deficiency after pregnancy, may have children that demonstrate symptoms of ADHD and various autism spectrum disorders. In my research, I have seen a connection between mother, child, and vitamin deficiency. As a result, you will notice that many of the anxiety and nervousness disorders related to vitamin B deficiency are also noted as similar symptoms and behaviors in the autism spectrum.

You will see many vitamin supplements on the market that contain 800 MCG a day or more in dosage of vitamin B12. Typically, when you take a vitamin supplement, your body will burn up the vitamins quickly due to stress. Your body uses only 25 MCG of vitamin B12 per day. Because the vitamin is so easy to burn off through stress, sweating, moving around, exercise, and other various scenarios, you will need to take a larger dose of the supplement. The best way to determine if you need a vitamin B12 supplement is not only by taking a blood test, but also by evaluating the foods that contain B vitamins to determine how much you are taking in.

Vitamin B12 deficiency is most often due to a defect in absorption. In many cases, vitamin B12 is not properly absorbed due to certain foods which block our stomach from absorbing it. For example, caffeine can deplete the body of vitamin B12, as well as of other vitamins. Although beer has some B vitamins in it, the levels are not really that significant. Alcohol is also a diuretic, and it causes loss of nutrients through the urine.

A 15-year-study on the effects of niacin (vitamin B3), published by the American Heart Association in the mid-1980s, connected the use of niacin to significant reduction in heart attack and death from heart disease. Long-term niacin use has been associated with decreased rates of cancer. Niacin should be taken under medical supervision, since it can also affect liver function.

Other B vitamins, such as folic acid and B12 can help lower blood levels of homocysteine, a risk factor for heart disease. Among the vitamins, vitamin B1 is the most important for the heart, so make sure your multivitamin contains 25 to 50 mg of it daily.

Many holistic providers take the approach to fortifying the system to prevent herpes outbreak. They state that antioxidants in the vitamins are the supplements that are important to people with herpes, since they both support immune function. On the B vitamin side, B6 and B12 are very important. I would recommend that the B vitamins should be taken in a combination or complex, as they work synergistically. Minerals, such as selenium and zinc, are particularly helpful in supporting the immune system in conjunction with using B vitamins.

Vitamin B12 has also been linked to infertility related to endometriosis (a condition in which the gland tissues that line the inside of the uterus grow outside the uterine wall), poor diet, iron deficiency, heavy metal toxicity, obesity, immature sex organs, abnormalities of the reproductive system, hormonal imbalances, and genetic damage from electromagnetic radiation. Several vitamin deficiencies, including vitamin B12, have been linked to the birth control pill. If a woman has been on the pill for a long time, she may be very low on folic acid, vitamins B1, B2, B6, B12, C, and E, and trace minerals such as magnesium, all essential to normal fertility.

Vitamin B deficiency has also been linked to lupus. According to Jonathan Wright, M.D., taking vitamin B6, up to 500 mg three times a day, will help relieve symptoms. People who live with this also need supplementation of hydrochloric acid.

Vitamin B12 deficiency has also been linked to multiple sclerosis. Multiple sclerosis patients generally have difficulty metabolically breaking down nutrients that they need for proper absorption of the vitamins into the body. Alcoholics, for example, can have the shakes, caused by the degeneration of their myelin, which is due to B12 deficiency. This seems very similar to the problems of multiple sclerosis. So, though a vitamin B12 deficiency is probably not the cause of multiple sclerosis, many people who suffer from this disorder have a B12 imbalance, one that doesn't necessarily show up on the blood test.

B12 deficiency is often missed for two reasons: it is not routinely tested by most physicians, and the low end of the laboratory reference range is too low. Thus, many people who suffer from B12 deficiency prove to have so-called "normal" levels of B12. The levels that are considered "normal" in the U.S. are between 200 pg/mL and 350 pg/mL. However, people with these levels have clear B12 deficiency symptoms. Many experts suggest treating all patients that are symptomatic and have B12 levels less than 450 pg/mL.

# 4. The Role of Methylcobalamin in Weight Loss and Fat Burning

## a) Obesity and Vitamin B12 Deficiency

In the human body we can differentiate three kinds of fat. The first kind is the structural fat, which is a sort of packing material that fills the gaps between various organs. Structural fat also performs important functions, such as cushioning the kidneys in soft elastic tissue, protecting the coronary arteries, and keeping the skin smooth and taut. It also provides the taut stress buffering cushion of hard fat under the bones of the feet, without which we would be unable to walk.

The second type of fat is a normal reserve of fuel upon which the body can freely draw when the nutritional assets from the intestinal tract is insufficient to meet the request. Such normal reserves are contained all over the body. Fat is a substance which packs the highest caloric value into the smallest space, so that normal reserves of fuel for muscular activity and the preservation of body temperature can be most carefully stored in this form. Both these types of fat, structural and reserve, are normal, and even if the body stocks them to capacity, this can never be called obesity.

But there is a third type of fat which is completely abnormal. It is the build-up of such fat and of such fat only, from which overweight people suffer. This abnormal fat is also a potential reserve of fuel, but, unlike the normal reserves, it is not available to the body in a nutritional emergency. It is, so to speak, locked away in a fixed "prison cell" and it's not stored in a place where it can easily be reduced in the same manner as the normal reserves.

When obese patients try to reduce this fat by starving themselves, they will first lose normal fat reserves. When these are depleted and patients begin to burn up structural fat, and only as a last resort, will the body release its abnormal reserves, though by that time people usually feel so weak and hungry that the diet is abandoned.

It is just for this reason that overweight people complain that when they diet they lose the wrong fat. They feel famished and tired, and their face becomes sunken and fatigued, and their belly, hips, thighs, and upper arms show little improvement. The fat they have come to detest stays on, and the fat they need to cover their bones gets less and less. Their skin wrinkles and they appear older. Wrinkles sag down, and frowning lines appear. That is one of the most infuriating and disappointing experiences a person can have.

Riboflavin (Vitamin B2) aids in the body's ability to burn flabby hanging fat in conjunction with a proper diet that is lower in sugar, carbohydrates, and caffeine. Also, Choline is a B vitamin that is a fat emulsifier in weight loss. It works in conjunction with Inositol. Choline and Inositol use the cholesterol and fats in the body to prevent weight gain and promote weight loss. Without Choline, the excess fats that are digested get collected in the liver, which leads to obesity.

## b) The Inheritance of Fat, and Diencephalic Illnesses

Let's take a look at the brain's diencephalic factor. The human diencephalon is comprised of several regions: the thalamus, which processes visual and auditory stimuli and generates some emotions among other functions, the hypothalamus, which has the primary pleasure center, regulates the autonomic nervous system, regulates the release of many hormones, regulates circadian rhythms, and determines many sexual dimorphic behaviors among other functions, and the pineal gland, which secretes melatonin and helps to generate circadian rhythms.

The diencephalon plays a role in your capacity to store fat. It follows the three basic ways in which obesity can manifest. The first is that the fat-banking capacity is abnormally low from birth. Such inherited low diencephalic ability would then represent the root reason of how one could explain how obesity can be inherited. When this abnormal trait is present, obesity will develop at an early age in spite of normal feeding. This could explain why among brothers and sisters eating the same food at the same table, some become obese and others do not.

The second way in which obesity can become recognized is the lowering of a previously normal fat-banking capacity owing to some other diencephalic disorder. It seems to be a general rule that when one of the many diencephalic areas is particularly overtaxed, it tries to increase its capacity at the expense of other centers. It robs one area of fat to compensate for an area that is losing fat.

In menopause or after having a hysterectomy, the hormones previously produced in the sex-glands no longer circulate in the body. In the presence of normally functioning sex-glands, the hormones halt, and the secretion of the sex-gland stimulating hormones of the anterior pituitary ceases. When drugs, or hormone creams, or various treatments jump start to get this going again, the anterior pituitary enormously increases its output of these sex-gland stimulating hormones though they are now no longer effective. In the absence of any response from the non-functioning or missing sex-glands there is nothing to stop the regulating and producing more and more of these hormones. This situation causes an excessive strain on the diencephalic center which controls the function of the anterior pituitary. In order to cope with this added burden, the center appears to draw more and more energy away from other centers, such as those concerned with emotional stability, the blood circulation (hot flashes), and other autonomous nervous regulations, particularly also from the not-so-vitally-important fat-bank.

After going through menopause and a hysterectomy, B12 deficiencies have been discovered. A maintenance dose of B12 needs to be taken daily to replenish the deficiency.

This can be looked at as being similar to what happens in the development of diabetes. It involves the diencephalic blood sugar regulating center (the hypothalamus), which tries to meet this abnormal load by switching energy destined for the fat-bank over to the sugar-regulating center, with the result that the fat-banking capacity is reduced to the point at which it is forced to establish a fixed deposit of storing fat, and initiates obesity.

In this case, one would have to consider diabetes as the primary trigger of obesity, but research has also shown that the process is reversed in a way where a deficient or overworked fat-center that is losing fat draws energy from the sugar-center. As a result, obesity would be the cause of diabetes. This is a type of diabetes that occurs when the pancreas is not primarily involved.

Finally, it is conceivable that in Cushing's Syndrome those symptoms which resemble obesity are also entirely due to the withdrawal of energy from one essential fat-bank and the anterior pituitary adrenocortical system (related to stress cortisol type belly fat), and draws fat into an area where it can be safely stored.

Whether obesity is caused by an inherited deficiency of the fat-center, or by some entirely different diencephalic regulatory disorder, its uprising obviously has nothing to do with overeating and, in either case, obesity is certain to develop regardless of dietary restrictions. In these cases, any enforced food deficit is made up from essential fat reserves and normal structural fat, which is much to the detriment of a person's health.

When cortisol is released in response to stress, an inflammation occurs. Elevated cortisol levels are associated with high homocysteine levels, an indicator of inflammation. Vitamin B12 (Methylcobalamin) helps regulate and reduce inflammation by converting homocysteine to methionine. In 2006, a study conducted by the *Clinical Chemistry and Laboratory Medicine* revealed that when serum B12 concentrations became exhausted, it was surmised that the effects of high cortisol on inflammation could be regulated by vitamin B12. You need to regulate a daily dose to aid in keeping the inflammation reduced.

## c) The Exhaustion of the Fat-bank

But there is still a third way in which obesity can occur. This can happen when a presumably normal fat-center is dealing with your overeating of an increased amount of food. At first glance, it does seem that here we have a straight-forward case of overeating being responsible for obesity, but on further research it becomes clear that the relation of cause and effect is not that simple. In the first place, we assume that the capacity of the fat center is normal, and we assume that people who have some inherited trait in this direction can become obese just by overeating.

Secondly, in many of these cases the amount of food eaten remains the same and your activity level changes. For example, when an athlete is confined to bed for many weeks with a broken bone, or when a person leading a highly active life is suddenly tied to their desk at work and to a TV screen at home. Another example is when a person grows up in a cold climate and moves to a tropical country, but continues to eat as before. This person may develop obesity because, in the heat, far less fuel is required to maintain the normal body temperature.

When a person suffers a long period of deprivation, be it due to chronic illness, poverty, famine or even war, this horrible situation causes them to decrease their food intake. When these conditions suddenly change, they are free to eat all the food they want, and this is liable to overwhelm their fat-regulating center. During wartime, when my family fled from India and relocated to Trinidad West Indies, many grossly underfed people who had spent their entire lives eating from a conservative diet of vegetables, fruit and rice were transferred to an island rich in beans, rice, chicken, beef, and many rich sugary foods, where they were well housed, given normal rations and some cash to buy a few extras. Within the first year, 85% were suffering from obesity.

In a person who eats coarse and unrefined food the digestion is slow and only a little nourishment at a time is assimilated from the intestinal tract. When such a person is suddenly able to obtain highly refined foods, such as sugar, white flour, butter, and oil, these are so rapidly digested and assimilated that the rush of incoming fuel which occurs at every meal may eventually overpower the diencephalic regulatory mechanisms, and thus lead to obesity. This is commonly seen in the poor man who suddenly becomes financially improved enough to buy the more expensive refined foods. Though his total caloric intake may remain the same or higher, he drastically replaced what he used to eat with foods that do not aid in weight loss.

## d) Vitamin B12 and Weight Loss

Recently, it has been discovered that there is a connection between vitamin B12 and weight loss. Even though B12 hasn't been proven to directly cause weight loss, it was noticed that it does contribute to the process by helping metabolize protein and fat. Well-metabolized protein and fat produce energy, and energy is one of the things that help people lose weight.

If you are trying to lose some pounds and you've decided to start exercising daily or a couple of times a week, then you know that sometimes it can be very difficult to motivate yourself. Usually, when that happens, the first reaction is to be disappointed with yourself because you feel like you aren't committed enough to your goal. But, before succumbing to these negative thoughts, ask yourself if the real problem isn't a vitamin deficiency. If your vitamin B12 levels are not adequate, then it's understandable that you lack the motivation and energy to go on with your diet and daily exercises. In this case, it is not your fault. All you need to do is to ask your health provider to run some tests, see what your body lacks in terms of vitamins and minerals, then choose those supplements that fit you best. And the first one to add to your diet is, of course, vitamin B12 in the form of methylcobalamin. It is fast, safe, and it will provide you with all the energy and enthusiasm you need to work out daily.

There are many reasons for which vitamin B12 is considered the best vitamin when it comes to weight loss. Knowing them is enough to understand why you should use it to support your healthy diet and your workout program. So, your body depends on vitamin B12 for a multitude of functions:

- It helps maintain normal energy levels.
- It is involved in the metabolism of carbohydrates and fats.
- It supports alertness and other neurological activities.
- It works with homocysteine levels for healthy heart function.
- It reduces stress and promotes sleep.
- It is involved in optimum immune function.

Many wellness clinics across the U.S. prescribe vitamin B12 injections because they speed up metabolism and help shed unwanted pounds. Injections work better than pills because you can see the effects sooner. The body absorbs the methylcobalamin quite fast, which means that you start feeling energized from the first couple of days of treatment.

# 5. Vitamin B12 Benefits the Nervous System

Vitamin B12 supports the health of your nervous system. In fact, research has shown that low levels of B12 cause peripheral and central nervous system damage that is linked to the onset of dementia and Alzheimer's disease. To get an idea of what this means, you need to know that the central nervous system governs the brain and spinal cord, while the peripheral nervous system presides over your body, face, arms, and legs.

Vitamin B12 is necessary for ridding the body of homocysteine, the substance that is associated with stroke and cardiovascular disease. It is also crucial in maintaining the integrity of the myelin sheath that covers the nerve fibers and allows for proper conduction of nerve impulses. The elderly are highly susceptible to vitamin B12 deficiency, which is caused by their inability to absorb vitamin B12. Reduced stomach acid, common in older people, leads to reduced absorption of vitamin B12. Deficiency of vitamin B12 at any age may lead to disorders of the nervous system.

Studies have proven that B12 helps in the healthy regulation of the nervous system, reducing depression, stress, and brain shrinkage. It maintains cardiovascular health, and regulates the cranial, spinal and peripheral nerves.

Let's see exactly what it does in case of different disorders that, unfortunately, are very common today.

## a) Anxiety and Depression

Anxiety and depression are two of the most common mental health concerns in our society. They are often experienced as a complex set of emotional and functional challenges, and even though they are not the same, they often occur together.

It is not uncommon for people with depression to experience anxiety, and for people with anxiety to become depressed.

Anxiety and depression may be triggered by a variety of factors which include nutritional, psychological, physical, emotional, environmental, social, and spiritual aspects, as well as genetic tendencies, or brain disease. There can also be a biochemical cause, meaning that certain chemicals in the brain, called neurotransmitters, are out of balance, and that can happen due to vitamin B12 deficiency.

Depression is a common disorder which currently affects over 350 million people worldwide. According to the Centers for Disease Control, one out of ten people report they have experienced a depressive episode. The disorder is typically characterized by low energy and mood, low self-esteem, and loss of interest or pleasure in normally enjoyable activities. The symptoms of depression include: sleep disorders, shifts in appetite and weight, irritability, chronic physical symptoms, such as pain, gastrointestinal disturbances, and headaches, loss of energy and fatigue, feelings of persistent sadness, guilt, hopelessness, or loss of self-worth, thinking difficulties, such as memory loss, challenges concentrating or making decisions, and even thoughts of death and suicide.

Anxiety, on the other hand, may be just a normal reaction to stress. However, when it becomes excessive, it turns into a disorder. The Anxiety and Depression Association of America estimates that almost one out of five people suffer from an anxiety disorder, which makes it the most common mental disorder in the United States.

Anxiety is characterized by emotional, physical, and behavioral symptoms which create an unpleasant feeling that is typically described using the words *uneasiness*, *fear*, or *worry*. The worry is frequently accompanied by physical symptoms, especially fatigue, headaches, muscle tension, muscle aches, difficulty swallowing, trembling, twitching, irritability, sweating, and hot flashes. Emotional symptoms include fear, racing thoughts, and a feeling of impending doom. People suffering from anxiety often withdraw and seek to avoid people or certain places.

A study published in 2010 in the *Journal of Orthomolecular Medicine*[1] showed how the treatment with intramuscular injections of vitamin B12 helped subjects who were complaining of idiopathic fatigue or tiredness. Even though they hadn't been diagnosed with vitamin B12 deficiency and their serum levels of vitamin B12 were normal, the study concluded that the intramuscular injections had a tonic effect. The subjects displayed a higher level of well-being and general happiness. They didn't feel tired or anxious anymore, and they were able to perform their daily activities with much more enthusiasm and determination.

The conclusion of this study was that the response to vitamin B12 was related to pharmacological factors, such as the ability of the vitamin to penetrate into the brain or neurons, or to an influence of vitamin B12 on neural metabolism.

Also, the study concluded that vitamin B12 can help patients who suffer from depression and anxiety because it lowers plasma and brain levels of homocysteine, which might mitigate, reverse, and potentially normalize, damaged brain neurons.

The same study presents two cases that demonstrate the benefits of maintaining high serum levels of vitamin B12. Both patients were suffering from anxiety symptoms, one of them having been diagnosed with severe depression coupled with obsessive-compulsive behaviors. After being on

---

[1] *Understanding the Serum Vitamin B12 Level and Its Implications for Treating Neuropsychiatric Conditions: An Orthomolecular Perspective*, Jonathan E. Prousky, ND, MSc Chief Naturopathic Medical Officer, Professor, Canadian College of Naturopathic Medicine; *Journal of Orthomolecular Medicine*. 2010;25(2):77–88 (http://www.townsendletter.com/FebMarch2011/b12psych0211.html).

antidepressants for years, they started a treatment with intramuscular injections of B12 (methylcobalamin and hydroxocobalamin), and in just a couple of months their conditions improved, allowing them to give up on the antidepressants. The injections with vitamin B12 improved their symptoms and helped them regain control of their lives.

## b) ADHD and Autism

It has been scientifically proven that methylcobalamin helps with ADHD symptoms through its involvement in many of the brain functions, especially in the production and maintenance of the myelin sheath, essential fatty acid metabolism, and energy production.

There is a strong link between vitamins and ADHD, because vitamins play an important role in the production of energy packets in the brain cells. Vitamin B12 is one of the most vital, because a B12 deficiency can hinder the production of energy, which might prompt the onset of ADHD. The disorder is characterized by hyperactivity, impulsivity, inattentiveness, and carelessness. It has been demonstrated that lack of sufficient vitamin B12 can lead to tiredness and depression, the two common symptoms associated with ADHD.

Dr. Richard A. Kunin has made extensive research on vitamin B12 and ADHD, and he has reached some interesting conclusions. First of all, he states that adenosyl-methionine can help in alleviating the patient's mood and mental sharpness. What vitamin B12 does is to join along with folic acid and work to ensure the maximum production of adenosyl-methionine. A sufficient quantity of B12 ensures the proper synthesis of S-adenosyl-methionine, thus promoting concentration, mental alertness, and a general feeling of well-being.

Moreover, Dr. John Lindebaum proved that lack of vitamin B12 can cause neurological troubles and a feeling of fatigue. A proper intake of vitamin B12 can help manage ADHD symptoms such as memory loss, depression, delusions, or difficulty in thinking. However, you must keep in mind that methylcobalamin cannot treat ADHD alone. It does reduce some of the symptoms of ADHD, but it cannot eradicate it completely.

In 2005, Dr. James Neubrander presented his discoveries related to the autism spectrum disorder and methylcobalamin at the Defeat Autism Now! conference[1]. In 2002 he had accidentally discovered that methylcobalamin had a positive effect on autism and other neurodevelopmental disorders, and in his presentation he outlined all the details.

One of the main benefits of methylcobalamin therapy is increased awareness. Soon after initiating this therapy, most children suddenly become more aware of their wants and needs. They are more aware of what they can and cannot do.

He reached the conclusion that the positive effects of methylcobalamin are predictable, reproducible, consistent, and undeniably obvious within the first five weeks of therapy. However, it is a treatment, not a cure. It has been proven that many children using methylcobalamin combined with other biomedical and non-biomedical therapies have lost their diagnosis, but the maximum results from this therapy occur over years. Though the initial results will be obvious within the first five weeks, methylcobalamin's power is in long-term use.

Dr. James Neubrander reported that 94% of children have been found to respond to methylcobalamin therapy. Executive function was improved in 90% of children – things like awareness, cognition, appropriateness, or eye contact when

---

[1] *Methyl-B12: A Treatment for ASD with Methylation Issues*; *Family Resources.* February 1, 2013 (http://www.tacanow.org/family-resources/methyl-b12-a-treatment-for-asd-with-methylation-issues).

called. Speech and language was improved in 80% of children – all phases including spontaneous language, more complex sentences, and increased vocabulary. Socialization and emotion was improved in 70% of the children – initiation and interactive play, understanding and feeling emotions, possibly for the first time or to a much more normal degree.

The effects of methylcobalamin are due to what it allows to happen in the brain, and what happens is that, in the presence of methionine synthase, methylcobalamin spins the methionine/homocysteine biochemical pinwheel, sending methyl groups and glutathione to the brain and body. In short, methylcobalamin allows the children to finally use the neurons and brain cells that have always been in place, but needed a boost.

Methylcobalamin has been proven to help children with methylation issues, and it can also help with some of the other issues that children on the autism spectrum can experience. Dr. James Neubrander used the treatment on his son, who is on the autism spectrum, and observed benefits in the following areas: additional speech, more complex sentence structures, he became more observant of his surroundings, better sleep patterns, better attention, and he gained a healthier complexion, and normal coloring was restored to his face.

## c) Short-Term Memory and Alzheimer's

Because vitamin B12 intake is necessary for healthy brain function, it is not surprising that a common cause for memory loss is B12 deficiency. We discussed the symptoms of this disorder in *Chapter 3*, and, as you can remember, they include memory loss and dementia. The Linus Pauling Institute notes that B12 deficiency increases the risk of high levels of homocysteine, which is linked to early onset of dementia and Alzheimer's disease.

A study conducted by Janine Walker, researcher at the Australian National University, has shown that adults who took vitamin B12 and folic acid supplements for two years had greater improvements on short and long-term memory tests than adults who did not take these vitamins. The results of the study were highly encouraging, proving that B12 has an important role in promoting healthy ageing and mental well-being.

Lowering homocysteine is important because the body uses it to build proteins, but high levels of it in the blood can cause heart disease, which is linked to mental decline. Methylcobalamin can help decrease the levels of homocysteine, thus ensuring a healthier heart and better cognitive functions.

Alzheimer's disease is the most severe form of dementia associated with memory loss. The risk of disease increases with age, and older people with low vitamin B12 levels are six times more likely to experience brain shrinkage, which is believed to be linked to the development of dementia. No cure has been discovered for this disease, which means that there's not much to do once the patient was diagnosed with it. It worsens as it progresses, the symptoms becoming more and more obvious. In the early stages, the common symptoms are short-term memory loss, confusion, and irritability. As the disease advances, the symptoms become more and more unpleasant and uncontrollable: aggression, mood swings, trouble with language, and, eventually, long-term memory loss. Alzheimer's is classified as a neurodegenerative disease, and its cause and progression have not yet been well understood.

Studies have shown that Alzheimer's disease is connected with vitamin B12 deficiency, and patients who suffer from this illness have lower serum B12 values compared to unaffected family members.

Vitamin B12 deficiency and its association with declining cognition have been studied for many years. Researchers discovered that deficient B12 levels correspond to both decline in cognitive ability, and a decrease in brain volume. Brain atrophy is a loss of cells that causes areas of the brain to become smaller, and it has been clearly identified as one of the physical effects of Alzheimer's disease.

An article in the *NY Times* shows how injections with vitamin B12 can have a positive effect on patients suffering from Alzheimer's[1]. An 87-year-old patient who was diagnosed with AD was also tested for vitamin B12 deficiency. Aside from prescribing medicines for Alzheimer's, the clinic also administered B12 injections to the patient on a weekly basis. Soon, the patient's memory and overall cognitive functioning dramatically improved.

A study has shown that a good way of preventing Alzheimer's disease is to reduce atrophy of key brain regions related to cognitive decline[2]. Thus, high-dose B12 treatment has been proven to reduce, by as much as seven fold, the cerebral atrophy in those gray matter regions specifically vulnerable to the AD process. The conducted study indicated that methylcobalamin lowers homocysteine, which directly leads to a decrease in gray matter atrophy, thereby slowing cognitive decline.

The conclusion is that once a patient was diagnosed with Alzheimer's disease, it is crucial to test him/her for vitamin B12 deficiency. Usually, the levels will be very low, and a treatment

[1] *It Could Be Old Age, or It Could Be Low B12*, Jane E. Brody; *The New York Times*. November 28, 2011 (http://www.nytimes.com/2011/11/29/health/vitamin-b12-deficiency-can-cause-symptoms-that-mimic-aging.html?_r=2&src=me&ref=general).
[2] *Preventing Alzheimer's Disease-Related Gray Matter Atrophy by B Vitamin Treatment*, Gwenaëlle Douaud, Helga Refsum, Celeste A. de Jager, Robin Jacoby, Thomas E. Nichols, Stephen M. Smith, and A. David Smith; Edited by Marcus E. Raichle, Washington University in St. Louis, St. Louis, MO, and approved March 29, 2013 (http://www.pnas.org/content/early/2013/05/16/1301816110).

with methylcobalamin can make a huge difference in how the disease progresses. It's true that currently Alzheimer's is untreatable, but methylcobalamin can, at least, show down its evolution and alleviate the nasty symptoms it causes.

## d) Pregnancy and Breastfeeding

Vitamin B12 deficiency during pregnancy and lactation may negatively affect fetal growth, brain development, pregnancy outcome, and breast milk vitamin B12 content.

Women who are trying to conceive, or are in their first trimester of pregnancy, are given folic acid supplements because research has shown that folic acid can help reduce the risk of the baby developing Neural Tube Defects (NTD), such as spina bifida, which can cause paralysis and anencephaly, a fatal condition in which the brain and skull are severely underdeveloped. However, new studies have come to the conclusion that taking vitamin B12 along with folic acid is even more effective. NTDs are birth defects of the brain and spinal cord that happen when the baby's neural tube fails to develop properly during pregnancy.

Women who have reduced levels of vitamin B12 are more at risk of having a baby with an NTD. This is why women should take folic acid and methylcobalamin supplements from three months before trying to conceive, while trying to conceive, and then for the first 12 weeks of their pregnancy, when the baby's central nervous system develops.

Vitamin B12 maintains normal folate metabolism, which is essential for cell multiplication.

Also, a study published in the journal Early Human Development in 2011 has shown how women who have low levels of vitamin B12 during their pregnancy have greater chances of giving birth to a baby with excessive crying behavior in the first months of life. On the other hand, women with high levels of B12 in their blood give birth to quieter babies. Researchers have suggested that excessive crying may be due to the fact that the baby's nervous system isn't fully developed, a problem caused by vitamin B12 deficiency during pregnancy. Also, a lack of B12 may reduce the brain's production of myelin, which is known to protect nerve cells, thus leading to more sleeplessness.

A high level of vitamin B12 is also beneficial for the mother during pregnancy, because it greatly improves her energy levels, and mood and stress levels. Future mothers who are deficient in B12 can suffer from fatigue, insomnia, anxiety, and even depression.

The reason why breastfeeding women have a higher need for vitamin B12 is that the developing fetus used a lot of the mother's stores of vitamin during pregnancy. A high level of B12 during breastfeeding is beneficial for both the mother and the baby. If ignored, a vitamin B12 deficiency can lead to serious problems, such as hematological, neurological, or gastrointestinal conditions.

As far as the baby is concerned, if he doesn't receive an adequate amount of vitamin B12 from breast milk, he may suffer from anemia, irritability, poor appetite, apathy, or developmental delays. At a later age, developmental regression, like impaired growth, gross motor function, poor school performance and other adaptive skills, has been suggested to be a consequence of a poor maternal vitamin B12 status during pregnancy[1].

The neonatal period is thought to be a special period of vulnerability to vitamin B12 deficiency.

---

[1] *Vitamin B12 in Pregnancy: Maternal and Fetal/Neonatal Effects – A Review*, H. Van Sande, Y. Jacquemyn, N. Karepouan, M. Ajaji; *Open Journal of Obstetrics and Gynecology*. 2013, 3, 599-602 (http://dx.doi.org/10.4236/ojog.2013.37107).

# 6. Healthy Sleep Patterns

The importance of quality sleep in the functioning of the human brain and body is absolutely crucial. Without it there can be severe psychological and physiological consequences. We all know that many physiologic processes occur during sleep, such as the increased secretion of growth hormone, enhanced immune function, and the scavenging of free radicals in the brain.

It has been estimated that 50% of the adult population is suffering from insomnia, with about 15% suffering from chronic insomnia, and 35% having transient or occasional insomnia.

As we've mentioned in the chapters dedicated to the symptoms of vitamin B12 deficiency, the lack of sufficient B12 in our system can also cause insomnia and depression. Vitamin B12 is closely connected with the hormone melatonin, which is responsible for regulating the circadian rhythms within our bodies. Melatonin regulates our sleep patterns. Thus, those who are suffering from B12 deficiency may experience altered sleep patterns, difficulty falling asleep, or lack of sleep because their bodies do not produce an adequate amount of melatonin.

According to the National Institutes of Health, the irregular sleep-wake syndrome is not that common. However, shift workers and the elderly may suffer from it. In the case of shift workers, this happens because they do not have a daily routine or a set schedule, and the fact that they often have to stay awake at night affects their circadian rhythm.

The circadian rhythm represents the physical, mental, and behavioral changes that come as a response to light and dark. The human body has a 24-hour internal clock which controls a number of processes, including the sleep-wake cycles. What causes the irregular sleep-wake syndrome is a near absence of the circadian rhythm that is responsible for regulating periods of wakefulness and rest.

People suffering from irregular sleep-wake syndrome usually sleep one to four hours at a time. The disorder is also characterized by excessive daytime sleepiness, restless nights, and frequent nighttime awakenings. Research has shown that methylcobalamin influences melatonin secretion, which means that a high level of vitamin B12 will increase the production of melatonin. Melatonin is a hormone produced by the pineal gland, and it is supposed to be secreted in higher amounts at night, when it is dark. It has been proven that methylcobalamin leads to improved sleep quality, increased day time alertness and concentration, and improved mood.

Methylcobalamin plays a major role in normal melatonin secretion. Low levels of melatonin, especially in the case of the elderly, may be a direct result of low vitamin B12. Several studies have shown that methylcobalamin is an effective treatment of sleep-wake disorders that are attributed to abnormal melatonin secretion.

# 7. How B12 Boosts the Effectiveness of Other Vitamins

## Using SAM-e and B Vitamins

Vitamin B12 is often used in vitamin B complex supplements that contain all the eight B vitamins. The reason why B complex supplements are highly recommended is obvious: the eight B vitamins work very well together, offering the body the energy it needs, and helping it convert food into fuel. Each B vitamin has its own role and they can, of course, be taken separately. Here is what each of them does:

**B1 (thiamine)** protects the immune system and helps the body produce new, healthy cells.

**B2 (riboflavin)** works as an antioxidant, prevents early aging and the development of heart disease, and it is also very important for the production of red blood cells.

**B3 (niacin)** boosts the good cholesterol, and studies have shown that it helps in the treatment of acne.

**B5 (pantothenic acid)** helps break down fats and carbs for energy, and it is responsible for the production of sex and stress-related hormones, including testosterone.

**B6 (pyridoxine)** helps the body produce serotonin, melatonin, and norepinephrine, which is a stress hormone. Along with vitamins 12 and 9, B6 helps regulate levels of the amino acid homocysteine.

**B7 (biotin)** is associated with healthy hair, skin, and nails. Also, it is very important during pregnancy because it's vital for the normal growth of the baby.

**B9 (folate)** helps in case of depression, and prevents memory loss. Together with B12, B9 supports the growth of the baby during pregnancy and prevents neurological birth defects.

**Vitamin B12 (cobalamin)** is considered a total team player, because it works well in combination with any other B vitamin. It boosts their effects.

B complex supplements are recommended for a variety of conditions, including anxiety, depression, fatigue, heart disease, premenstrual syndrome, and skin problems. However, they can also be taken when you're not suffering from any of the above, but you consider that you'd benefit from increased energy, enhanced mood, improved memory, and a stronger immune system.

Vitamins B9 and B12 are essential for the normal development and function of the central nervous system. The metabolism of these vitamins is intimately linked and supports the synthesis of S-adenosylmethionine (SAM-e), the major methyl group donor in methylation reactions.

First, let's talk a bit about SAM-e, and try to understand what it is and what it does. S-adenosylmethionine is a naturally occurring compound that is found in almost every tissue and fluid in the body, and it is made from the essential amino acid methionine and adenosine triphosphate (ATP). SAM-e works as a methyl group donor in many reactions in the body, and after it donates the methyl group, it is converted to a compound called S-adenosyl-homocysteine.

SAM-e plays an important role in the immune system, it maintains cell membranes, and helps produce and break down brain chemicals, such as serotonin, melatonin, and dopamine. It works very well with vitamin B12 and vitamin B9. Actually, if you are deficient in either of these two vitamins, then you also have reduced levels of SAM-e. Vitamin B12 participates in the production of SAM-e and, therefore, it plays a decisive role in the functioning of the neuropsychiatric system. An adequate production of SAM-e facilitates the formation of phospholipids that comprise neuronal myelin sheaths and cell receptors, and the synthesis of monoamine neurotransmitters. Insufficient vitamin B12 would decrease the production of SAM-e, which would impair methylation and, consequently, impair the metabolism of neurotransmitters, phospholipids, myelin, and receptors.

SAM-e was first discovered in Italy, in 1952, and it has been available as a dietary supplement in the U.S. since 1999. Now, SAM-e is used for many health problems because it has been scientifically proven that it treats pain, stiffness, and swelling of the joints. Moreover, it improves mobility, it rebuilds cartilage and relieves osteoarthritis symptoms, it relieves chronic low back pain, and it helps in treating depression. Let's look more closely at SAM-e's effects when used to treat some of the disorders mentioned above.

## Osteoarthritis

Clinical trials have shown that SAM-e reduces pain and inflammation in the joints, and promotes cartilage repair. It seems to be just as effective as non-steroidal anti-inflammatory drugs, which are prescribed to patients suffering from knee, hip, or spine osteoarthritis. Thus, it lessens morning stiffness, decreases pain, reduces swelling, improves range of motion, and increases the walking pace, everything with fewer side effects than non-steroidal anti-inflammatory drugs.

## Depression

It has been proven that SAM-e can help treat depression just as effectively as antidepressant medications, without the side effects. Moreover, SAM-e shows results more quickly than antidepressants, and this adds greatly to the advantage that patients don't have to suffer from the headaches, sleeplessness, and sexual dysfunction caused by antidepressants. The reason why SAM-e works so well for depression is that it can raise levels of several brain chemicals, including norepinephrine, serotonin, and dopamine.

## Liver Disease

SAM-e helps treat chronic liver disease caused by medications or alcoholism, and it has been proven that taking SAM-e for two years can improve survival rates, and delay the need for liver transplants in the case of people suffering from alcoholic liver cirrhosis. People with liver disease cannot synthesize SAM-e in their bodies, and what SAM-e does is to normalize levels of liver enzymes. It can protect against liver damage, and it may even reverse it.

Asides from the diseases mentioned above, SAM-e may also be used for anxiety, heart disease, fibromyalgia, dementia, Alzheimer's disease, chronic fatigue syndrome, and Parkinson's disease. However, people taking SAM-e are strongly advised to take a multivitamin that contains B12 and B6 to reduce its side effects, which can include restlessness, headaches, and insomnia, but only if it is taken in higher doses.

Patients who intend to take SAM-e need to be aware that it may interact negatively with certain medications, and they should first consult their health care provider. SAM-e shouldn't be taken with pharmaceutical antidepressants or dietary supplements that have a stimulating nature due to their quality of increasing serotonin in the brain. This combination may lead to headaches, irregular or accelerated heart rate, anxiety, restlessness, and even to the fatal condition called Serotonin Syndrome (too much serotonin in your body). Also, it may interact with medications for diabetes because it reduces the levels of blood sugar and strengthens the effect of the treatment, which may lead to an increased risk of hypoglycemia.

Studies haven't yet discovered the effects of SAM-e in pregnant and breastfeeding women, but they are strongly advised to avoid taking it during these periods.

# 8. B12's Role in Improving Diabetes Mellitus

Diabetes mellitus, also known as simply diabetes, is a group of metabolic diseases caused by high blood sugar levels. Untreated, diabetes can lead to long-term complications, such as heart disease, stroke, kidney failure, or damage to the eyes.

This serious disorder is related to insulin: either the pancreas does not produce enough of it, or the cells of the body do not respond properly to the insulin produced. The three main types of diabetes mellitus are:

Type 1 DM – The body fails to produce enough insulin.

Type 2 DM – Cells fail to respond to insulin properly, thus causing insulin resistance. The primary cause of this type of diabetes is excessive body weight and not enough exercise.

Gestational Diabetes – It occurs when pregnant women without a previous history of diabetes develop a high blood glucose level.

It has been estimated that 382 million people have diabetes worldwide, with type 2 diabetes making up about 90% of the cases. It is the 8th leading cause of death, which was proven by the fact that in 2012 and 2013 diabetes resulted in 1.5 to 5.1 million deaths per year worldwide. It is a dangerous disease that can, at least, double the risk of death even when treated properly.

Researchers have noticed that clinical and biochemical vitamin B12 deficiency is highly prevalent among patients with type 1 and type 2 diabetes[1]. There are various reasons for which this happens.

---

[1] *Vitamin B12 Deficiency Among Patients with Diabetes Mellitus: Is Routine Screening and Supplementation Justified?*, Davis Kibirige, Raymond Mwebaze;

In case of type 1 DM, the patients actively exhibit auto antibodies to intrinsic factor, and parietal cell antibodies. The parietal cell antibodies inhibit the secretion of intrinsic factor, thus leading to pernicious anemia. Vitamin B12 deficiency occurs frequently among patients with type 1 DM.

Cross sectional studies and case reports have documented an increased frequency of vitamin B12 deficiency among type 2 DM patients. It has been proven that metformin, which is the first-line drug of choice for the treatment of type 2 DM, decreases vitamin B12 levels by 22% and 29% as a side effect. The risk of developing metformin associated vitamin B12 deficiency is greatly influenced by increasing age, metformin dose, and duration of use.

Because both types of diabetes attack the intrinsic factor and interfere with the absorption of B12, it is a good idea to at least perform screenings for vitamin B12 deficiency. If the disorder is present, then B12 supplementation is necessary to increase the vitamin's levels and promote better health.

Also, patients suffering from diabetic retinopathy might consider taking a vitamin B complex. Diabetic retinopathy is a complication that causes damage to the blood vessels in the eye, and it is directly linked to increased blood levels of homocysteine. Vitamin B12 lowers those levels and improves the disorder, which affects up to 80% of all patients who have had diabetes for 10 years of more, and even threatens to lead to blindness if it is not treated properly.

In case of diabetic neuropathy, which is a painful nerve damage that afflicts the legs and feet, B12 has been proven to minimize symptoms such as pain, numbness, prickling, and tingling.

*Journal of Diabetes and Metabolic Disorders.* 2013; 12:17 (http://www.ncbi.nlm.nih.gov/pmc/articles/PMC3649932).

I decided to write this section on diabetes and diabetic neuropathy because, over the past three generations, I've seen many family members suffer from pain from diabetic neuropathy, and also from degenerative eye disorders and retinal detachment.

The sad thing for me is hearing the cries of pain, and it is that kind of pain that feels like it is constantly stabbing and will not let up. A constant zapping pain in the feet and hands, and it's as if you can feel your blood vessels breaking. One of the turning points for me in researching vitamin B12 and its effectiveness was being able to give sublingual vitamin B12 (Methylcobalamin 1,000mcg) drops to family members to help with blood vessel supplementation.

One of the things I noticed was that my relatives displayed the ability to buffer daily stress more easily. Previously, they would feel a heightened sense of tension and agitation when their diabetic medication or insulin would be starting to work its release into the body. They could sense the stress that you feel when the blood sugar is dropping or raising. Supplementing with vitamin B12 aided in achieving increased emotional stability while decreasing depression and agitation.

Taking vitamin B12 can improve the disposition to feeling dizzy, which is often common in case of a low carbohydrate diet. Typically, when I hear anyone seeking intervention for diabetes, I ask them to consider that their condition is not only diabetes, but also malabsorption.

Vitamin B12 is best taken sublingually, as a liquid drop under the tongue, for fast absorption. Hard caps that melt under the tongue are also available, yet, at the end of the day, you want to know that you received the fastest and most effective mode of delivery. So, test it out and see if you prefer a liquid or a hard capsule.

Some diabetics can also have asthma. When taking B12, it can strengthen the lung function aiding in alleviating the symptoms of asthma. Some diabetics who have asthma get triggered by certain foods, so I recommend that you research foods that are high in sulfites and try to notice if they trigger episodes. If they do, eliminate them from your diet.

New research shows success in diabetes management, especially in balancing the nervous system and metabolic system. Because it energizes the body, B12 relieves fatigue, depression, and poor concentration. A vitamin B12 deficiency can take five or more years to appear after the body stores have been depleted. Deficiency results in anemia, nervous system degeneration, dizziness and heart palpitations, and it contributes to unhealthy weight loss in diabetics. Sometimes, diabetics can feel dizzy, they can feel their heart palpitating, and they think their blood sugar is dropping. When they check their glucose level, they realize it is not the case. What may be low is their Vitamin B levels, which can give them similar symptoms. Long-term use of various prescription drugs, such as cholesterol-lowering drugs, oral contraceptives, anti-inflammatory and anticonvulsant drugs, may also deplete vitamin B12.

Vitamin B12 helps bolster energy, and aids those suffering from type 2 DM to properly use the insulin they produce effectively in their body to convert food into energy glucose. Otherwise, the insulin tends to build up in the bloodstream, and they can't absorb the nutrients they need. Supplementation with vitamin B12 accelerates the absorption of vitamins and nutrients.

When researching alternative health references for nutritional intervention related to diabetes, you tend to see similar advice recommending a low carbohydrate diet, and several herbs and supplements that treat the symptoms of diabetes, such as cinnamon, selenium, chromium picolinate, nopal cactus, and apple cider vinegar.

Another nutritional intervention that is used to help with neuropathic pain includes alpha lipoic acid and omega-3 oils. You need to really monitor your blood glucose level when taking alpha lipoic acid and omega-3 oils because it can severely drop your blood sugar. I advise taking it two hours before you take your medication or insulin, and seeing how low your blood sugar drops. Discuss with your medical provider about adjusting your dosage to accommodate that lowered glucose reading.

When seeking to balance healthy blood sugar through nutritional intake, you cannot ignore the importance of vitamin B12 vitamin. It helps the utilization of many vitamins, including iron, and it is required for the proper digestion and absorption of food. You have to understand that when you suffer from diabetes, your goal is to be able to properly utilize and break down complex sugars and carbohydrates in food.

In addition, having diabetes long-term is linked to nerve pain and damage. Vitamin B12 aids in healthy cell formation and cellular longevity. It also promotes and protects the nervous system by maintaining the protective fatty sheath coating around the nerve endings.

# 9. What is Methylation? What Kind of Methylator Are You?

Methylation is the process of controlled transfer of a methyl group onto amino acids, proteins, enzymes, and DNA in every cell and tissue of the body to regulate healing, cell energy, genetic expression of DNA, neurological function, liver detoxification, immunity, etc. Actually, we can say that it is a key biochemical process that is essential for the proper functioning of almost all body's systems. Methylation occurs billions of time every second, it helps repair the DNA on a daily basis, it controls homocysteine, and it helps recycle molecules needed for detoxification. If methylation isn't running smoothly in your body, there's an increased risk of developing some serious diseases, such as chronic fatigue syndrome, autism, heart disease, depression, sleep disorders, or dementia.

The process of methylation requires two cycles of events: the SAM-e cycle, and the folate cycle. It depends on a number of vitamins and cofactors which must be present for adequate functioning. The absolutely necessary vitamins are B9 and B12. To keep methylation running smoothly, you need optimal levels of B vitamins, because without them methylation breaks down, and the results can be more than unpleasant. This kind of breakdown can put you at higher risk for osteoporosis, diabetes, depression, stroke, and even cancer. To avoid all these problems, you only need to make sure that your methylation is normal. But, first of all, you have to figure out what kind of methylator you are: a hypomethylator, or a hypermethylator. If none of these two categories apply to you, then it means that your methylation processes are optimal, and you only need to keep them that way through a proper diet.

A hypomethylator has poor methylation processes, which means that the person is suffering from a decrease in levels of serotonin, dopamine, and norepinephrine. To normalize your methylation processes, you need to increase these levels, and you can do that with the help of methionine, SAM-e, magnesium, calcium, zinc, and vitamin B6. Hypomethylators reacts poorly to folic acid and vitamin B12.

Hypermethylators are usually prone to anxiety, hyperactivity, or obsessive compulsion disorder. This can be explained by the fact that they have high methylation processes, high levels of dopamine and norepinephrine, and low levels of folic acid and vitamin B12. In order to decrease methylation, you can take supplements of folic acid, as well as vitamins B12, B5, and B3.

There are many factors that can affect the methylation process, and some of them can be controlled quite easily by maintaining a healthy diet. A poor diet that does not include leafy greens, beans, fruit, and whole grains can affect your levels of vitamins B6, B9, and B12. On the other hand, a diet that is high on animal protein, sugar, saturated fat, coffee, and alcohol can raise the levels of homocysteine and deplete the B vitamins. Smoking is known to inactivate vitamin B6, and certain medications can also affect the levels of B vitamins – acid blockers, methotrexate (for cancer and arthritis), oral contraceptives, and medications for high blood pressure and seizures. Decreased stomach acid can also lower the absorption of vitamin B12, as well as any other digestive diseases. Unfortunately, genetics may be involved as well, and we know that there's nothing that can really be done about it. Studies have shown that 20% of people are genetically predisposed to high homocysteine.

# 10. Vitamin B12 Deficiency and Its Trigger in Illness and Disease

As we have discussed in *Chapter 3*, vitamin B12 deficiency can cause permanent damage to nervous tissue if left untreated for longer than 6 months. It can even become fatal, and the bad news is that the nerve deterioration can continue if the treatment is not adequate or is interrupted at a certain point. This is why it is important to pay attention to symptoms that might indicate that you are suffering from B12 deficiency, because it is crucial to discover it early and start treating it. Failing to do so can lead to some serious complications, such as megaloblastic anemia. Cardiovascular diseases are also connected to vitamin B12 deficiency, because low levels of B12 in the body lead to high levels of homocysteine, which have been proven to be a risk factor for cardiovascular disease, blood clotting abnormalities, atherosclerosis, heart attack, and stroke. Also, B12 supplements have been shown to reduce the risk of adverse cardiac events after the performance of coronary angioplasty. Moreover, some evidence has shown that B12 supplements may prevent cancer. This theory is supported by the fact that patients suffering from cancer usually have low levels of vitamin B12 in their blood.

## a) Megaloblastic Anemia

We already know that vitamin B12 deficiency causes pernicious anemia, which is an autoimmune disease in which the body's own autoimmune system damages its own tissues. Pernicious anemia is actually a form of megaloblastic anemia, which refers to an abnormally large type of red blood cell called megaloblast. Megaloblasts are produced in the bone marrow, when vitamin B12 and folic acid levels are low. It is a disorder caused by incomplete formation of the red blood cells, which eventually results in large numbers of immature and incompletely developed cells. These red blood cells do not function like healthy blood cells, and crowd out the healthy cells, thus causing anemia.

The main cause of megaloblastic anemia is vitamin B12 deficiency. The body lacks proper levels of B12 due to the deficient absorption of the vitamin, and this leads to pernicious anemia. However, megaloblastic anemia can also be caused by other problems, such as alcohol abuse, chemotherapy, leukemia, certain medications, or even some genetic conditions.

The most common symptoms of megaloblastic anemia are: fatigue, muscle weakness, loss of appetite, undesired weight loss, diarrhea, nausea, fast heartbeat, tingling in hands and feet, numbness in extremities.

When treating megaloblastic anemia, many aspects will be taken into consideration. The doctor will first establish the underlying reasons for the anemia, then he/she will make a prescription based on the patient's age, overall health, the severity of the disease, and the tolerance and response to treatments. Of course, if the main cause of the anemia is a general lack of vitamin B12 in the body, then the prescription will probably involve monthly injections of the vitamin. Also, a healthy diet that is rich in eggs, meat, poultry, milk, and shellfish will help a lot, because these foods contain a lot of B12 and folic acid.

## b) Angioplasty and Cardiovascular Disorders

Many studies have suggested that people with high levels of the amino acid homocysteine are more likely to develop coronary artery disease and have a stroke, than those with normal levels. There is a strong connection between blood homocysteine levels and heart disease risk proven by a number of observational studies that have found that people with low homocysteine levels had a lower incidence of heart disease than people with higher levels of homocysteine. Naturally, vitamins B6, B9, and B12 keep homocysteine at a relatively low level in the body, but when the absorption of these vitamins is hindered, the levels rise and the person is in danger of developing heart disease.

It was clearly demonstrated that giving extra amounts of B12 lowers homocysteine levels, thus reducing the risk of cardiovascular disease. However, vitamin B12 deficiency is not what causes cardiovascular disorders directly. It is true that it contributes to the development of these diseases, and makes people more prone to them, but the causes of cardiovascular disorders are diverse, atherosclerosis and hypertension being the most common. The risk factors are also quite diverse: age, gender, high blood pressure, diabetes mellitus, smoking, excessive alcohol consumption, obesity, lack of physical activity, and even psychosocial factors.

There are many types of cardiovascular disorders, each manifesting in different ways. I'm only going to mention some of them: coronary artery disease, cardiomyopathy, cardiac dysrhythmias, cerebrovascular disease, peripheral arterial disease, congenital heart disease, rheumatic heart disease.

Patients who have undergone angioplasty might also want to take some B12 supplements at least six months after the procedure. Angioplasty is the technique of mechanically widening narrowed or obstructed arteries, and it is generally used in the treatment of atherosclerosis and coronary heart disease. After the intervention, patients are advised to avoid physical activities for at least a week, but the recovery is not as simple as it may seem. There is a major problem that remains after using angioplasty in the treatment of coronary artery disease: the risk to develop restenosis.

Restenosis is a common adverse event of angioplasty that consists of the narrowing of a blood vessel after it was widened with the help of a balloon. In cardiac procedures, for instance, balloon angioplasty has been associated with a high incidence of restenosis, almost half of the patients needing a further angioplasty within only six months. Because high levels of homocysteine are a risk factor for heart disease, we also know that after angioplasty they become a risk factor for restenosis. A study published in the Journal of the American Medical Association has shown that a 6-month regimen of B vitamins aimed at reducing homocysteine levels can significantly lower the risk of restenosis after angioplasty.

## c) Cancer

A number of research studies covering types of cancer such as colon, stomach, or breast cancer have linked the disease to lowered levels of vitamin B12. It seems that vitamin B12 deficiency can be one of the causes of cancer, given that it has been noticed that patients suffering from a form of cancer tend to have low levels of B12 in their blood. But this is not all. The worst part is that chemotherapy and surgery employ drugs and antibiotics that can reduce the digestion and the absorption of vitamin B12 even more. Naturally, this means that supplementation with B12 and other B vitamins, including folic acid, is crucial for patients who are suffering from any form of cancer.

Another problem is that most patients decide to change their diet as part of their personal cancer therapy program, and they often become vegan or vegetarian. Because vitamin B12 can only be found in products that come from animals, they actually manage to do more harm to themselves by further lowering their levels of B12. This can have terrible consequences, especially if their cancer was associated with vitamin B12 deficiency in the first place. Fortunately, there is a solution for these patients who choose to change their diets, and that solution is methylcobalamin.

A study has shown that methylcobalamin can reduce the tumor growth and enhance survival time in patients suffering from cancer or leukemia. On the other hand, cyanocobalamin has proven to be completely ineffective. Methylcobalamin can protect the organism against cancer thanks to its ability to donate a methyl group, and thanks to its role in the regeneration of SAM-e, the body's universal methyl donor.

# 11. Hormonal Balance and Methylcobalamin. My Personal Journey

After my first pregnancy I became over 70 pounds overweight. I felt depressed and tired all the time. My chiropractor had an on-site lab at his office, and advised that I take a blood test to determine if my iron was still up. I was diagnosed with low iron during my pregnancy, and my family doctor had previously advised me to take an over-the-counter iron available, an OTC called *SLow Fe*. I tried it, but soon I realized that I just didn't feel right. I couldn't think straight, and I was angry, upset and moody all the time. It didn't help the fact that I was also nursing, and that made me feel very weak and gave me a constant raving appetite.

After taking an updated blood test after my pregnancy, my chiropractor told me that not only was my iron low, but my levels of vitamin B12 were also severely low. He was the one who educated me about the relationship between vitamin B12 and iron. He recommended taking over-the-counter nutritional iron liquid called Floradix, a product that is made in Germany but is widely available at many health food stores in the United States. In addition, he also recommended taking sublingual vitamin B12 drops, more specifically, methylcobalamin, due to it being a more naturally occurring form of B12. After taking these supplements for two weeks in conjunction with maintaining my prenatal vitamins, I noticed a tremendous turnaround in my emotional well-being, my energy and endurance to get through the day. Previously, I had also been unable to produce enough lactation for nursing. After being on the B12 and iron, I personally noticed (although I had not seen research to back up what I was witnessing) a better balancing of my vitamin levels, and an increase in normal and healthy lactation.

You would think that after going through all of that I would maintain healthy habits. I didn't. I went off the vitamin regimen when I was done nursing, and years later I was diagnosed with high blood pressure. I became frightened when I literally had a menstrual cycle for 3 months straight, and I found out that conventional medicine only offered surgical solutions. What I did was contact a provider of saliva and hormonal testing at Sabre Sciences in California. This is how I found out that I was what was called a *hypermethylator*, which meant that the regular B vitamins which contain cyanocobalamin were causing by body to retain water. They were also causing me to bleed severely.

As I have explained at the beginning of this book, cyanocobalamin leaves a cyanide residue in the blood stream. It is often used in regular B vitamins and in OTC multi-vitamins. The best option was to use the methylcobalamin form of Vitamin B12, so I started using it in a transdermal crème, and I still do. The purpose of using the crème is for the vitamins to go right into the blood stream by bypassing the liver, in order to help heal the adrenal glands. After much more research, I also found out about the oral benefits of taking B-complete, which works very well in full vitamin B absorption, without the side effects of traditional vitamin B.

My ability to handle stress has improved, and now I still monitor my blood pressure level daily because I remember the previous torture of feeling the stabbing headaches that came with the increase of my blood pressure. I supplement taking B12 with L-Arginine and Omega 3 to maintain healthy blood pressure levels. In a recent PBS educational series on heart health, Dr. Brenda Watson recommends taking Celery Seed and Hawthorne Extract. B12 has made a difference in my life by helping me maintain my weight loss. A good B12 supplement will also contain Riboflavin, which aids in the burning of hanging flab when used in conjunction with a low carb diet.

I'm sharing my story with you to encourage you to research your missing link. If you feel like you have had similar ailments or symptoms listed anywhere in this book, I implore you to research your vitamin deficiencies. Ask your trusted health provider to test your vitamin levels. I have also mentioned in this book that your vitamin B level can be low even if it doesn't show up in a blood test. Check your dosages in your multi-vitamin supplements and ask your health provider about the recommended daily dosages that will work best for you.

In this respect, you must know that there are two types of allowances. There is a recommended daily allowance (RDA), which was instituted over 40 years ago by the U.S. Food and Nutrition Board as a standard for daily amounts of vitamins needed by a healthy person. Unfortunately, the amount they came up with give us only the bare minimum required to ward off deficiency diseases, such as beriberi, rickets, scurvy, and night blindness. What they do not account for are the amounts needed to maintain maximum health, rather than borderline health.

Scientific studies have shown that larger doses of vitamins help our bodies work better. The RDA, therefore, is not useful in determining what our intake of different vitamins should be. I prefer to speak in terms of optimal daily allowance (ODA) – the amount of nutrients needed for vibrant good health.

By providing our bodies with an optimum daily allowance of necessary vitamins, we can enhance our health. The dosages that I'm about to outline will enable you to design a vitamin dosage that you can research and discuss with your trusted health provider. Please keep in mind that B vitamins should always be taken together, because they work as a team. A vitamin B12 complex will typically contain a blend of: vitamin B2 (riboflavin), vitamin B3 (niacin), vitamin B6 (pyridoxine HCL), vitamin B12 (methylcobalamin), folic acid, vitamin B5 (pantothenate).

The optimal daily allowance (ODA) should be researched carefully and discussed with your trusted health provider:

An ODA B12 Vitamin Drops Dosage Range:

- vitamin B2 (riboflavin) 1.7 to 2 mg;
- vitamin B3 (niacin) 20- 25 mg;
- vitamin B6 (pyridoxine HCL) 2mg - 5mg;
- vitamin B12 (methylcobalamin) 800mcg- 1200mcg;
- folic acid 400mcg;
- vitamin B5 (pantothenate) 30mg - 40mg.

# 12. Dosage Recommendations, Safety, Drug and Supplement Interactions

The doses recommended in this chapter may not apply to all patients, disorders, or even products. They are meant to offer you some guidance, even though they are based on scientific research, publications, traditional use, or expert opinion. It comes without saying that you should read product labels and discuss doses with a qualified health care provider before starting therapy.

For children (under 18 years old), the adequate intake (AI) levels of vitamin B12 are as follows:

For infants 0-6 months old: 0.4 micrograms (AI);
For infants 7-12 months old: 0.5 micrograms (AI);
For children 1-3 years old: 0.9 micrograms;
For children 4-8 years old: 1.2 micrograms;
For children 9-13 years old: 1.8 micrograms.

For adults (18 years and older), the recommended dietary amounts (RDAs) are as follows:

For ages 14 years and older: 2.4 micrograms daily;
For pregnant women: 2.6 micrograms daily;
For breastfeeding women: 2.8 micrograms daily;
For people over 50: supplementation of 25-100 micrograms daily.

For vitamin B12 deficiency, the following doses will be given intravenously: 1,000 micrograms of intramuscular cobalamin once daily for 10 days. After 10 days, the dose is changed to once weekly for four weeks, followed by once monthly for life.

For prevention of anemia, the following doses need to be taken by mouth: 2-10 micrograms of vitamin B12 daily combined with iron and/or folic acid for up to 16 weeks; 100

micrograms of vitamin B12 every other week, plus daily folic acid and/or iron for up to 12 weeks.

For depression, the recommended dose is one milligram of cobalamin through intramuscular injections, weekly for four weeks.

Before you decide to begin therapy with vitamin B12, you should speak to your health care provider, especially if you are taking other drugs, herbs, or supplements. Moreover, B12 supplements might have side effects in case of certain health conditions, so if you're suffering from one of the following, you should use them cautiously.

- Allergies – B12 supplements should be avoided by people who are allergic to B12, cobalt, or any other product ingredient;
- Heart concerns;
- High blood pressure;
- A history of cancer;
- Skin disorders;
- Gastrointestinal concerns;
- Blood disorders.

It also has to be used cautiously in people taking the following agents, as they have been associated with reduced absorption or reduced serum levels of B12: ACE inhibitors, acetylsalicylic acid, alcohol, antibiotics, anti-seizure agents, bile acid sequestrants, chloramphenicol, colchicine, H2 blockers, metformin, neomycin, nicotine, nitrous axide, oral contraceptives, para-aminosalicylic acid, potassium chloride, proton pump inhibitors, tobacco, vitamin C, and zidovudine.

# RESOURCE INDEX

- http://www.todayhealthnews.info/p/vitamin-b-12-for-diet.html
- http://www.todayhealthnews.info/2011/10/b12-1000-mcg-methylcobalamin.html
- http://www.raysahelian.com/sam-e.html
- http://www.ncbi.nlm.nih.gov/pubmed?uid=10459691&cmd=showdetailview&indexed=google
- http://www.ncbi.nlm.nih.gov/pmc/articles/PMC3888748
- http://www.ncbi.nlm.nih.gov/pmc/articles/PMC3649932
- http://toothwiz.com/wordpress/?p=251
- http://www.mayoclinic.org/drugs-supplements/vitamin-b12/evidence/HRB-20060243
- http://www.mayoclinic.org/drugs-supplements/vitamin-b12/dosing/hrb-20060243
- http://www.mayoclinic.org/drugs-supplements/vitamin-b12/safety/hrb-20060243
- http://www.mayoclinic.org/drugs-supplements/vitamin-b12/interactions/hrb-20060243
- http://www.tacanow.org/family-resources/methyl-b12-a-treatment-for-asd-with-methylation-issues
- http://www.livestrong.com/article/454179-what-is-methyl-b12
- http://www.ncbi.nlm.nih.gov/pubmed/23651730
- http://www.dadamo.com/B2blogs/blogs/index.php/2004/02/07/cyanocobalamin-versus-methylcobalamin?blog=27
- http://www.aafp.org/afp/2003/0301/p979.html
- http://www.townsendletter.com/FebMarch2011/b12psych0211.html
- http://www.natural-alternative-adhd-treatment.com/vitaminb12.html
- http://www.progressivehealth.com/vitamin-b12-adhd.htm

- http://www.nytimes.com/2011/11/29/health/vitamin-b12-deficiency-can-cause-symptoms-that-mimic-aging.html?_r=2&src=me&ref=general
- http://www.pnas.org/content/early/2013/05/16/1301816110
- http://www.nutraingredients.com/Research/Vitamin-B12-in-pregnancy-could-lead-to-quieter-babies-Study
- http://advances.nutrition.org/content/3/3/362.full
- http://www.healthline.com/health/irregular-sleep-wake-syndrome
- http://doctormurray.com/health-conditions/insomnia-sleep-wake-cycle-disorder
- http://bioclinicnaturals.com/ca/en/articles/4/conditions-and-diseases/7/sleepwake-disorders/show/18/insomnia-and-sleepwake-cycle-disorders
- http://umm.edu/health/medical/altmed/supplement/sadenosylmethionine
- http://www.webmd.com/vitamins-supplements/ingredientmono-786-SAMe.aspx?activeIngredientId=786&activeIngredientName=SAMe
- http://altmedicine.about.com/od/treatmentsfromatod/a/SAMe.htm
- http://osteoarthritis.about.com/od/alternativetreatments/a/sam-e.htm
- http://www.enzymestuff.com/methylation.htm
- http://drhyman.com/blog/2011/02/08/maximizing-methylation-the-key-to-healthy-aging-2
- http://www.hdri-usa.com/assets/files/role_of_b_vitamins_in_biological_methylation.pdf
- http://heartdisease.about.com/library/weekly/aa090202a.htm
- http://www.thebetterhealthstore.com/news/VitaminB120601.html

- http://www.canceractive.com/cancer-active-page-link.aspx?n=513
- http://goodshape.net/B12Thorne.html
- *"Demystifying Weight Loss: A Concise Guide for Solving the Weight Loss Puzzle"*, Pamela Wartian Smith, M.D., MPH
- Beth Masters, http://lapappaorganics.com Researcher

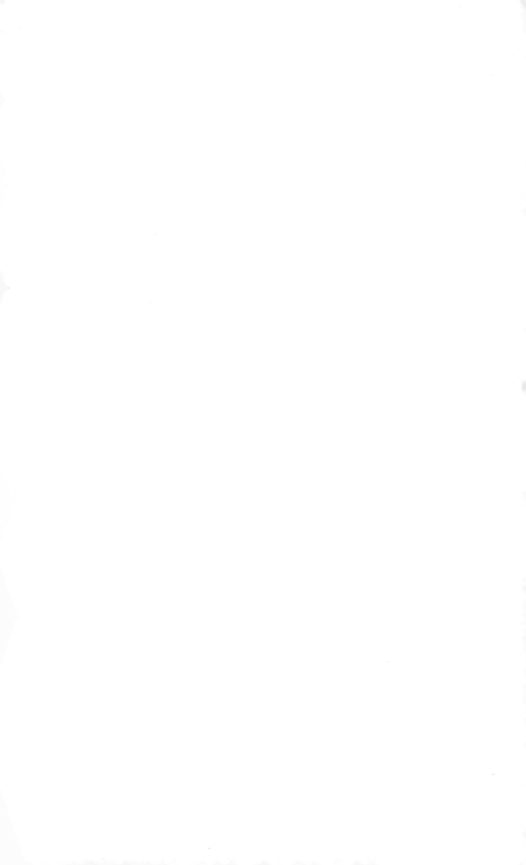

23540628R00041

Printed in Great Britain
by Amazon